THE ULTIMATE GUIDE TO WORKING FROM HOME

THE
ULTIMATE GUIDE TO WORKING FROM HOME

**STAY SANE, HEALTHY AND
MORE PRODUCTIVE THAN EVER**

GRACE PAUL

sphere

SPHERE

First published in Great Britain in 2020 by Sphere

1 3 5 7 9 10 8 6 4 2

A CIP catalogue record for this book is available from the British Library.

Ebook ISBN 978-0-7515-8149-2
Hardback ISBN 978-0-7515-8150-8

Typeset in Garamond by M Rules
Printed and bound in Great Britain by Clays Ltd, Elcograf S.p.A.

Papers used by Sphere are from well-managed forests
and other responsible sources.

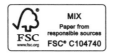

Sphere
An imprint of
Little, Brown Book Group
Carmelite House
50 Victoria Embankment
London EC4Y 0DZ

An Hachette UK Company
www.hachette.co.uk

www.littlebrown.co.uk

CONTENTS

PART THREE: LOOKING AFTER YOURSELF

PART FOUR: IT'S NOT ALWAYS EASY

PART FIVE: MAKING WORK WORK FOR YOU

CONCLUSION: WHAT THE FUTURE HOLDS

INTRODUCTION

So you may have decided to take the plunge and start working from home, or you might be curious about it. Maybe you've gone freelance, you've taken up your employer's offer of flexible working, or redundancy has forced you to change your work practices. Either way, you're not alone.

By the end of 2019, one in five[1] of us around the globe were already working from home before so many more of us were forced to due to coronavirus. Getting started and understanding what works best for you can feel overwhelming because there's just so much information out there, but fear not: you're in the right hands. As someone who used to work for a multi-million-pound corporation in an office and has been navigating the ups and downs of working from home since going freelance, I've written the guide I wish I'd had.

The way we work is constantly evolving. There's been a 74 per cent increase in those who work from home since 2008, with over 1.5 million people[2] in the UK alone now enjoying the benefits and flexibility that this way of working can offer. According to a survey by the Association of Independent Professionals and the Self-employed (IPSE), over half[3] of the respondents said flexibility was the greatest advantage for them when it comes to working from home. However, working from home doesn't just benefit employees, it also benefits employers and businesses. In a survey conducted by the International Workplace Group (IWG), eight out of ten[4] businesses said that flexible working has made their business more productive. In fact, working from home is one of the fastest growing employment benefits companies offer new employees. Done well, it often enables staff to have a better quality of life and businesses can save money.

Most of those who are seasoned at working from home will tell you that the key to their success is setting a daily routine, establishing boundaries and looking after their mental and physical well-being. This book will show you how to implement these important strategies, and more besides.

But what about when your routine isn't working for you, you're feeling your motivation ebb away, you don't know how to talk to your manager about it or you have to share your space with others? We'll cover all of that, too.

To help you, I've divided this book into five parts:

Part One – Why work from home: in this section, we'll look at the myriad reasons why working from home is beneficial to both you and your employer (if you have one).

Part Two – Working well: in this part, we'll explain how you should set up your home office; how to organise yourself so you're the most productive you can be, and how to communicate effectively.

Part Three – Looking after yourself: we'll look at how you can set yourself up in your home, create boundaries when it comes to your work-life balance, and look after your mental and physical health.

Part Four – It's not always easy: in this section, we discuss how to work when others are at home – be it your partner, children or housemates – and what to do when you simply cannot find your working from home mojo.

Part Five – Making work work for you: we'll look at how you can best speak to your manager or team about working from home so you can equip yourself with the tools you need to ensure success. Plus we'll look towards the future of working from home.

You should dip in and out as you please to find the answers you're looking for. Feel free to navigate this book in exactly the way that works for you – just like you'll learn to do with your own working life.

PART ONE

WHY WORK FROM HOME?

Nicholas Bloom, a Stanford University economist, has described working from home as having as much potential as a driverless car[5]. This might sound like a big claim, but there's an overwhelming wealth of evidence to back it up, from the impact working from home has on the planet to our mental well-being. So, let's look at some of the key aspects of home-working.

The upsides of working from home

Economy

You may think that working from home will only save *you* money but it will, in fact, save money for your employers, too. Firstly, you could save over £1,500 a year on lunches, as the average officer worker spends over £6[6] a day on lunch. And then there are your commute costs. In America, on average, a worker can spend between $2,000-5000[7] a year on getting to and from the workplace. Though this isn't as bad as cities such as London, Sydney and Dublin, which are currently the top three most expensive commutes in the world[8]. The average UK employee spends £146 on their monthly commute. Think of what else you could do with that money by the time you retire. And then there's the amount of time you spend commuting – the average UK worker spends 400 days[9] of their lives doing so. As we all know, you can't put a price on time.

So how do employers benefit from their staff working from home? Running an office space is a huge expense – the average cost for a square foot of office space in London, for example, costs seventy pounds a month[10], and in Manchester it costs about thirty pounds[11]. Then there's staff retention. We all know that having a happier team means fewer members of staff leave. In fact, the average cost of hiring a new employee is £11,000, based on someone earning an average salary of around £28,000[12]. This includes the obvious stuff but also the many hidden costs including the time invested by staff in the hiring phase, onboarding paperwork and the deferred productivity of the new team member as they learn the ropes. Working from home is a recognised staff incentive and British, American, Australian and Indian businesses (among others) all use working from home flexibility as a way to attract and retain staff. In Poland, 92 per cent[13] of employers use this strategy and German and Belgian workers are more likely to reject a job if work flexibility isn't an option.

Diversity

Offering employees the option to work from home opens up the door for those unable to work in an office full time because of health, personal circumstances (such as carer responsibilities), age or disability. This means that home working can increase the workforce talent pool.

For example, working from home is hugely important for those with a disability – over a million[14] disabled people work from home. It is also hugely beneficial when it comes to parents returning to the workforce after parental leave as it allows a far better chance of being able to juggle childcare and a career. By allowing parents to be more flexible, companies can help close the gender pay gap by allowing women to continue with their career. Despite the fact that women remain the principal carers for children, you may be surprised to hear that it's still almost twice as many men[15] as women who work from home.

Disappointingly, those from a BAME background are less likely to be able to work from home compared to white workers – 4.3 per cent to 6.5 per cent[16]. This may be because BAME millennials are 47 per cent[17] more likely than white millennials to be on a zero-hours contract and 5 per cent more likely to do shift work which means that they're unable to do their job at home. According to the Trade Unions Congress (TUC), this is most probably because decisions can be disproportionality made on the basis of job title hierarchy[18]. Managers are twice as likely to work at home compared to the average employee, with nearly one in eight managers doing so on a regular basis[19].

Enabling people to work from home means that you can tap into talent anywhere in the country, or even the world, as someone's job role isn't dependent on their location. By doing this, workforces will be more diverse and, in the long run, more financially beneficial. In 2017, management consulting firm McKinsey & Company did a survey with over 300 companies worldwide and those who were in the bottom quartile for both gender and cultural diversity were a third less[20] likely to achieve above-average profitability compared to their more diverse counterparts.

Productivity and happiness

FlexJobs ran a survey with 3,000 people in 2018[21] and over two thirds of those who took part said that working from home has allowed them to be happier due to flexibility in their life. Interestingly, 65 per cent said they were more productive, too. It's not too much of a leap to suggest that happier staff get more done. According to a study by Prithwiraj Choudhury, an associate professor in the Technology and Operations Management Unit at Harvard Business School, this productivity gain could add $1.3 billion[22] to the US economy every year.

Then there's the dreaded commute. A study about commuting and well-being from the University of the West of England (UWE) has found that job satisfaction declines with commute time[23]. In fact, the study noted that an additional twenty minutes of commuting each day could 'have the equivalent effect on job satisfaction as a 19 per cent reduction in income.' In the

UK, the average commute time is fifty-nine minutes, which equates to 221 hours a year. Imagine how much happier we'd feel if we ditched the commute.

Health

Your mental and physical health is going to thank you for working from home, especially as you won't be commuting every day. You'll be able to use this extra time to do exercise more regularly or spend extra time with your family, which will have an effect on your overall well-being. Plus you're not going to be exposed to everyone's germs in the office. In fact, those who work from home are only sick 1.8 days a year compared to workers in an office who take an average of 3.1 sick days[24].

Environment

Commuting not only puts a strain on us individually, it also has a big impact on our planet.

The car is the most used mode of transport for commuting, with just over half[25] of British workers travelling to work in this way. Seeing as the average worker in the UK spends over an hour commuting, imagine how much carbon dioxide is being pumped into the atmosphere. In fact, in London, a car costs the NHS and society £8,000 in health bills due to air pollution[26]. If a quarter of car journeys were spent walking or cycling, then the nation could save over £1.1bn a year[27]. Not only is this wrecking our health but it's a major contributor to climate change.

But are you really working as hard as your office-based counterparts?

We all know someone who enjoys working from home on a Friday so they can take it easy. Perhaps you've been guilty of it yourself. I know I have. If you do a quick Google search for working from home, the images that come up will be of people in their pyjamas, someone holding a baby whilst on a work call, working in bed – they don't paint the best picture.

These working from home myths aren't actually as solid as you think they are. In fact, the opposite may be true. According to a study of 16,000 employees working at a Chinese travel agency, conducted by Stanford University professor Nicholas Bloom, productivity increases by well over 10 per cent[28] when people work from home, partly because there are fewer distractions and they work longer hours. Gig economy company Airtasker polled over a thousand people across the US, half of whom worked in an office, about their efficiency in the workspace. On average, those who worked from home worked an extra 1.4 days a month and sixteen days a year[29], leading to financial gain for their employer. So the next time someone says to you that only slackers work from home, feel free to quote these facts.

PART TWO

WORKING WELL

You might think that working from home simply consists of sitting down with your laptop and getting on with it but there are a lot more factors to take into consideration. Do you know how to behave on work virtual calls? How are you going to avoid 'tech neck'? And are you allowed to reward yourself with food? (the answer is always yes on that last one).

Creating the right set-up for you

According to a study carried out by the office equipment firm Fellowes[30], a quarter of workers said they had pain caused by a poor home office set-up and this impacted their productivity. Having the right set-up is beneficial for both the employer and employee and you have no excuses not to prioritise it.

The average office worker spends 1,700 hours[31] at their desk a year, so it's important to get this right. The main thing to remember is that your set-up needs to be ergonomic, meaning that the equipment and furniture you use is as comfortable and effective as possible so you can perform your job to maximum efficiency without causing your body any permanent damage. Matthew Devoe, an American chiropractor, explains that a bad set-up will likely result in 'tech neck'[32], which consists of headaches and spasms caused by hunching over your desk too much. This is easily avoided if you do the following:

- Your keyboard and mouse, or keypad, should be level with or below your elbows.
- Elevate your laptop, if using one, to ensure that the screen is at eye height, using a separate monitor or keyboard as necessary.
- Rest both feet on the floor or on a footrest.

You can also complete a DSE, a display screen equipment assessment, which will help you assess your home office and identify any risks or hazards that might affect your health. You can readily download a DSE for free, I recommend looking up The Health and Safety Executive (HSE)'s website.

Desk

The right desk for you will depend on the space you have. You may be fortunate enough to have a separate room to act as your home office, or you may be living in a small bedroom in a house share, or alternatively you might only have one table in your home. Fear not, you can always make your space work for you, however small it is.

In an ideal world, you'll have a designated desk or table that you can work at. If you have a limited space, why not contemplate getting a foldable desk or a cardboard desk, such as the one available from cardboard furniture company aiBox. If you only have one table in your house, I suggest finding a way to use it differently in work mode and in home mode. This can be as simple as turning your table around so it faces the wall during the day and at the end of your working day, moving it so you're facing out to the room. Packing up your desk and work tools at the end of the day is also a great way to switch from work to home mode – you might not have a door you can shut on your workspace, but you can put it all in a cupboard so it's out of sight.

We know that sitting all day isn't good for our bodies so how about trying a standing desk? The British Journal of Sports[33] highly recommends this as good for your physical health and your productivity levels, reducing the number of sick days you need to take. If you're unsure about going straight to a standing desk, you can buy a height adjustable one so you can sit and stand.

The most important thing about working at a desk though is to get up every hour and move around for a few minutes. The brain works better when we move, instead of spending hours hunched over our desk, as the blood flow to our brain increases which leads our productivity to grow as a result[34].

Chair

Ideally, you'll be able to get an ergonomic desk chair which is adjustable and preferably reclines as this will reduce the strain on your neck. The opportunities are endless when it comes to office chairs, as is the price range, so have a look online for one that suits your needs best. If you don't know where to begin, you could try calling a reputable office furniture company and their trained staff will be able to guide you through the ideal set-up for you, or you could speak to a qualified DSE assessor.

If you don't have the space or the budget for an office chair to use at home, you can get creative. Ellen Kolber, founder of ErgonomicsNYC[35], says that placing a pillow on your chair, be it a foldable chair or a dining table one, will elevate you and relieve pressure on your spine. Remember that your chair is the only thing between you and the hard floor, so it is an important investment.

Lighting

Lighting is an important factor when setting up your own home office as it will ensure you remain alert, boost productivity and reduce eye strain. Eye strain is caused by excessive light, be it sunlight coming in through the window or harsh indoor lighting, so this is the most important thing to keep an eye on in your home workspace. Symptoms include sore eyes, blurred vision, eye-twitching or headaches. To avoid this, according to Specsavers opticians[36], reduce the glare of outside light by drawing the curtains or blinds, and indoor lighting by using a desk or floor lamp instead of harsh overhead lighting. If you're using a lamp, the best option is one with a dimmer, so the light is softer and less intense. You should also adjust your screen brightness to as low a level as you can use whilst still being able to see things clearly. You can also invert the colours on your screen, so the background is black and the text is white. Additionally, you should position your screen at least 51cm[37] away from your eyes as the closer they are, the harder they have to work to focus.

What technology will you need?

Now that you've got your physical space set up, you need to ensure that you have the right gear so you can do your job as efficiently as possible. Technology has revolutionised working from home and continues to do so by offering faster and better ways of connecting remotely. Even so, four out of ten[38] workers in the UK still say that a lack of necessary technology provided by their employer prevents them from working from home as often as they'd like. You might be able to afford your own equipment or make a case to your employer to provide you with the technology you need. Read on to learn how you can make technology work for you.

Screen

Ideally you'll be able to use a desk-top computer rather than a laptop – desktops have more power, a longer life and are normally easier to set up at the correct height. They also have a more powerful fan so they're less prone to overheating. A top tip I had to learn the hard way – working on a laptop in bed fries the insides of a laptop as the soft duvet cover blocks all airflow through the machine.

If you are unable to use a desk-top, because of cost, lack of availability or space, you can look into getting a monitor to use in conjunction with your laptop. They are readily available and more affordable than they used to be so they're worth considering if they suit your needs.

If you don't have a desk-top or a monitor, you could also consider a separate keyboard (see below) and an elevated laptop. You might look into a cardboard frame or a laptop stand that allows you to place your laptop and keyboard at the appropriate heights. Worst case scenario, I would suggest using a stack of books to prop your screen up to the correct height for you. This is the most readily available and economical option.

Keyboard and mouse

As mentioned, the crucial aspect of a good ergonomic home office set-up is elevating your screen so it's at eye height to avoid straining your neck. To do this, you'll preferably have a separate keyboard and mouse. If you're happy to use a touchpad then good for you but for others a mouse is essential, especially a wireless one. Make sure you have a good mouse pad as a piece of paper just isn't going to cut it!

If you can't get a keyboard or if you don't have the space to accommodate one, an adjustable laptop stand is a good alternative. These tip the back of the laptop up by a couple of inches to raise the screen but keep the keyboard accessible.

Headphones

I cannot deny that listening to good music increases my productivity and mood tenfold and I'm not alone. American firm Cloud Music conducted a survey of one thousand people[39] and almost half of them reported using headphones to avoid distractions whilst 80 per cent of them said that using headphones helped boost their productivity.

One of the main complaints of working in an office is the constant distractions. You may be working from home now, but there can still be plenty of distractions and not only if you happen to share your space with other people. Headphones can help you get in the zone, which is also perfect if you live on your own and can easily find ways to distract yourself. If you have the budget, I suggest noise-cancelling headphones; not only will they drown everything out, but they'll be handy to use when video calling clients or colleagues as well. You may also want to consider using a headset if the quality of your device's sound and volume aren't sufficient and you want to avoid sounding echoey on a call.

You might not want to listen to music but you may miss

the general chatter of working in an office. Check out the website www.asoftmurmur.com which provides an array of ambient sounds to help you avoid distractions.

Software and internet

What equipment do you need for your job? You might be a journalist who needs transcribing software or a banker who needs stock-trading software. Assess what you need and discuss with your employer if you need their help getting set up.

You will also need to consider cyber and data security, as cyber-crime is on the rise. As such, your company may require you to have certain confidentiality software installed as well as encrypting your devices. Encryption software will lock your files and data away with a code meaning that only authorised personnel can access it, therefore avoiding it falling into the wrong hands. You can protect your data by setting up your devices with encryption software such as BitLocker (Windows) or FileVault 2 (Mac). If you work for a company, your work server should automatically back up your work but I would also recommend backing up onto a hard drive to be on the safe side. We've all felt that existential dread when our computer crashes in the middle of a task, so do what you can to avoid it.

Finally, it goes without saying that if you're working from home, then you're going to need a good internet connection. Speak to your provider about data limits to ensure you have enough capacity to be as effective as possible.

Communication

You may wonder why there's a section in this book about how to communicate with others, especially virtually. I think we've all seen the BBC footage from 2017[40], which has been viewed by millions of people, when Professor Kelly was gatecrashed by his children during a live interview he was doing with the broadcaster. Here are some top tips:

Dress appropriately: not having to wear a suit is one advantage of working from home, but it shouldn't be an excuse for staying in your pyjamas all day. There is a happy medium to be had. Dress comfortably day to day and if you are doing a video call with colleagues or clients who are office-based, consider dressing more formally, not least so that you convey an aura of professionalism. It's like when you have a day with no external meetings and the next day you have to give a presentation to a client, you dress accordingly for physical meetings, so incorporate that into your working from home attire as well.

Turn up on time: if you're having a meeting on the phone or online, make sure you're on time just like you would be in a physical meeting. Speaking from experience, it is just as irritating to be kept waiting in a call room as it is to be kept waiting in a meeting room.

Mute yourself when you're not talking: OWLLab's 2019 State of Remote Work[41] report found that interruptions and being talked over are two of the biggest meeting challenges for both remote and on-site workers, so don't be that person.

Don't try to multitask: be present in the meeting instead of trying to answer other emails whilst you're on a call. We all think we're fantastic at multitasking but the truth is we are not (actually only a measly 3 per cent[42] of us are any good at it) plus it's rude, particularly when people can see you on video. Stick to one thing at a time.

Let's get to work

We all know that organisation is the key to productivity – it's as old as time, yet still we struggle to sit down and focus. Discovering what works for you is very empowering and once you've cracked it, you'll notice a real difference. The steps below should set you on the right path.

Creating the right routine for you

Make your own rules but, for the love of God, if you possibly can, do set a work routine and a post-work routine as this will keep you sane.

Set your schedule: decide what your working days and hours are and tell those you work with. Not only will this help you be more productive, but it will also help you set boundaries with the rest of your team or clients.

Write a to-do list: this will help you remain focused and motivated during the day. Personally, I get a real sense of achievement when I tick tasks off as I go. See the to-do list section for more on how to make your to-do list work for you.

Breaks: make sure you have regular breaks, including a lunch break and a tea break, just like you would if you were working in an office.

Get outside: leave the house and get some fresh air as it will help break up your day and boost your energy. If you can't leave your house or don't have any outside space, move away from your desk and open the windows to allow some fresh air in.

Stay connected with others: working from home may make you feel excluded from the rest of the world so arrange plans for after work, be it in person or virtually. For the latter, you can install apps on your devices such as FaceTime, Houseparty and Zoom.

Mark the end of your day: according to a survey by online brand development agency Buffer, the biggest working from home complaint is being unable to unplug at the end of the day. Kristen Shockley, an associate professor of psychology at the University of Georgia, suggests 'psychological segues'[43] such as a coffee or a workout to close your working day. Set a small ritual – whatever it takes to tell your brain it's no longer work time.

To-do list

We assume that a to-do list consists of jotting down a long list of the tasks you need to complete that day and getting on with it. However, according to life coach Rachida Benamar[44], we make the mistake of writing everything down without any structure. For example, you might find yourself writing 'get milk' next to 'write presentation for work'. By doing this, you are likely to find yourself overwhelmed or unable to focus on the tasks on hand. Here's how to create the most effective list:

Priorities: your performance targets and deadlines should determine your priorities for the day so remember to take a look at the bigger picture instead of focusing on minute details.

Structure: Rachida recommends putting your three most important tasks at the top of your list and aiming to do them first. By doing your most important tasks first, you'll feel a sense of achievement which in turn will boost your mood for the rest of the day. If you can keep your to-do list to under five items, then all the better as this way you'll avoid feeling overwhelmed and more motivated about what you have to achieve during your working day. By incorporating this structure into your list, as well as adding in time blocks for tasks, you'll avoid getting frustrated and wasting time. When you're scheduling in your time blocks, bear in mind when you're at your most productive in the day so you can dedicate that time block to the tasks that require your thought and focus. Create time blocks for tasks that don't require all your brain power, such as admin, emails and follow-up phone calls, when you're feeling less productive. If you're unsure about how long a task should take you, consider speaking to your manager or colleagues for advice.

Get a calendar: logging your deadlines and tasks into a calendar, be it digitally, on a wall calendar or in a journal, will make your work feel more real. Enter your deadlines with a note a few days before to tell you the deadline is coming up.

Time Management

Working from home doesn't mean working non-stop without any breaks. You may struggle keeping your mind focused so you need to learn about how and when you work best.

Firstly, are you an early bird or a night owl? Sleep specialist and author of *The Power of When* Michael Breus[45] has discovered that there are four types of people in the world, depending on their sleep habits. By discovering your sleep type, you'll be able to take advantage of your body's natural energy flows and discover when you're at your most productive during the working day. The four categories are: bears (50–55 per cent of the population with a morning routine of 7–11 a.m., consisting of what you do before work such as brushing your teeth, having breakfast, etc., followed by peak work hours of 11 a.m. to 6 p.m.), lions (15 per cent of the population, who get up between 5:30–10 a.m., typically when it's dark outside, and whose peak work hours are 9 a.m. to 5p.m.), wolves (15–20 per cent of the population who hit the snooze button and get up between 7:30 a.m. and 12 p.m., with peak productivity between 12 and 8 p.m.) and dolphins (1 in 10 of us have sleep problems and their morning routine is between 6–10 a.m with peak productivity between 10 a.m. and 6 p.m.). Working out when you work best will help ensure peak productivity. In case you're wondering, I'm a bear mixed with a bit of wolf as I work best in the evening.

This is all well and good but how do you keep your mind focused for a set amount of time? Clifford Nass, a professor of communication at Stanford University, did a study on cognitive control in multitaskers[46]. The results led him to suggest that we should spend at least twenty minutes focusing on one task instead of flitting between many different ones. To keep your mind on the task at hand, there are a wide array of time management techniques out there.

I've tried a few approaches and can highly recommend the Pomodoro Technique, named after a tomato-shaped egg timer. The technique was developed in the 1980s by Francesco Cirillo and is particularly useful for project-based work or for when you want to dedicate a certain amount of time to reactive tasks such as answering emails or dealing with inbound issues. Decide what task you want to focus on, set a timer for twenty-five minutes, then work on the task. Once the timer has gone off, take a three- to five-minute break then set your timer for another twenty-five minutes and repeat. After you've done this four times, take a longer break of fifteen to thirty minutes. There are a wide range of free apps (see useful tools on pp. 67) which you can set up on your devices that will automatically run the timer for you.

If this doesn't sound right for you, you could create a smart playlist[47] that changes songs at set intervals, e.g. two minutes for each email, so you maintain your momentum. It doesn't take long to set up and it's surprisingly effective.

Hygiene

Yes, really. Whatever you do, even when you're having a bad workday, wash, brush your teeth, brush your hair and get dressed. It will have a big impact on your mood and help you separate your work life from your home life. American psych- ologists[48] discovered that wearing more formal clothing can boost your abstract thinking – the ability to think about the bigger picture surrounding an event or idea. Whilst another study[49] revealed that wearing a doctor's coat can help you be more focused. So next time you decide to wear your pyjamas for a day's work, perhaps think about how much this might affect your productivity.

Avoid distractions

We live in a society where we're constantly distracted by technology and notifications. If you want to be as productive as possible, draw up a list of the main things that distract you: for example, television, phone, household chores, and make sure you stay away from them wherever possible. Turn off your notifications on your phone and stop social media for blocks of time with an app such as SelfControl, available on either your phone or desktop.

Rewards

Rewarding yourself when you've completed a task, especially a difficult one, is very valuable when working from home. To boost motivation, set up a rewards system for yourself: I would suggest one of your favourite distractions, going for a walk, having lunch with a friend, eating your favourite bar of chocolate, or you could go wild and give yourself the afternoon off.

Motivation

The right set-up, a daily routine and a robust rewards system will all contribute to your sense of motivation. Sometimes though, no matter what you do, it's just not happening.

You might think that changing your mindset when it comes

to motivation isn't possible but it really is a psychological thing. If you change your mindset about the project you're working on then you can make things easier for yourself. Psychologists have identified three key elements[50] that sustain your motivation:

Autonomy: your current mindset might be 'I have to do this' and feeling as if you're being forced isn't going to help you. Instead flip your mindset to 'I choose to do this' and remind yourself that you have the autonomy to do this task on your own. You're choosing to do your work because it has a positive effect on your life: financially, mentally and socially.

Value: when lack of motivation is taking hold, ask yourself what value working from home is bringing to your life. It might be that the value of it is purely financial, or it might be because it's a stepping stone to the next stage in your career or even going for a mid-morning swim. Whatever it is, the task you're doing is beneficial to your life so bear that in mind.

Competence: sometimes we find ourselves trying to do a new piece of work and exclaiming, 'I can't do this'. Remember that you *can* do it but the first time is always the hardest. The more you flex a certain work muscle, the stronger it will get.

Whenever your motivation is flagging, take a step back and work out why this is happening. Chances are you can flip it on its head to get yourself back in the zone.

PART THREE

LOOKING AFTER YOURSELF

You may be working from home because you have others to care for, for financial reasons or because you're more productive in a home environment. Whatever your reasons are, you need to look after yourself so you're as sharp, motivated and as healthy as you can be. Work and home life both feed into each other, so self-care is of paramount importance.

Work-life balance

We know that businesses are using flexible working as a way to improve their employees' work-life balance[51]. Sometimes, though, those who work from home struggle with drawing the line between work and life, leading to them working longer hours overall. An American online branding agency did a survey and the participants' biggest struggle with working from home was being unable to unplug from work[52]. Women have it harder, according to research published in 2019 by the Hans Böckler Foundation in Germany.

Whilst working from home enables more flexibility for parents, it can also mean three hours[53] of extra childcare per week which typically falls on women. However, it is possible to create the right work-life balance by following a few simple steps – some of these have already come up in the productivity section but they're useful when it comes to boundary setting as well:

Set clear working hours: make sure your team, clients and family are aware of these and make sure you stick to them.

A designated workspace: this way you'll be able to switch from home to work mode, plus this will send a signal to others as well.

Hobbies: having something set in the diary will ensure that you don't miss out on hobbies. Working from home makes it too easy to prioritise finishing a job over activities like taking a walk, going for a swim, going to the gym or meeting friends. Schedule these in as part of your routine and stick to them.

How to stay sane

Whilst working from home tends to be many people's dream set-up, it is easy to underestimate how the shift from an office to a home office will impact you mentally. Loneliness is the top culprit – who knew you could miss those office kitchen chats with Sharon so much?

Stay connected

When I first started working from home, I cannot deny that I found the loneliness crippling. I've now found what works for me to keep it at bay: hobbies (such as playing the guitar and flailing around in yoga classes) and plans with friends in the evening. This won't be right for everyone but it's important to find out what works best for you.

An American brand agency [54] did a study with 2,500 remote workers in 2019 and loneliness was the second-most reported challenge after unplugging from work.

So what can you do to vary your schedule to get what you need socially?

Get out of the house: the joy of working from home is the flexibility it gives you to enjoy the rest of your life. Why not go out for a walk or a run or even to a gym class at a time when you know it isn't going to be busy?

Stay connected: try and start the day with a phone or video call so you're connected with the outside world and you can switch better into work mode. Emails help but speaking to someone will help even more.

Switch it up: you may only be working from home a couple of days a week or you may be working from home full-time, but if you have the option of a laptop it does give you the option to mix things up in terms of location. Why not look into a co-working space (you can rent a desk hourly or daily in most spaces) or join one of the many online communities on MeetUp, Facebook or Coworking Map, a website that lets you view co-working spaces all over the world. You might even change where you work in the house if you're not inclined or able to go out.

Go to events: attend networking events, either virtually or in person. Not only will they be beneficial from a work perspective but you will meet others who can understand the challenges you may be facing and can sympathise with how you feel.

Mental well-being

Looking after your mind is key, especially if you find yourself alone a lot more than usual now you're working from home. Working out and getting outside plays a big part in your mental well-being, as does practising mindfulness. It helps you focus on the present and reduce stress and anxiety which may be induced by work. Fortunately, working from home means that you can use what would have been your commute time to add extra activities into your life. The following tips can help you calm your mind:

Breathing exercises: one of the quickest and most effective ways to calm a racing mind. Breathe in through your nose for four seconds then exhale out of your nose for eight seconds. Repeat for up to three minutes and notice the sense of stillness you feel afterwards.

Scan through your body: when was the last time you checked in with your body and how you really feel? Sit down and close your eyes. Starting from the top of your head, scan down through your body paying attention to how you feel, noting any tension or strong emotions. Don't be hard on yourself for what you find, it's simply good to know what's going on in our bodies and minds.

Meditation: check out apps such as Headspace and Calm to help you find a little bit of peace during your busy everyday life.

How to look after your body

Physical well-being

Whilst working from home allows more flexibility overall, it can also lead to a more sedentary life as the walk from your bed to your desk and to the fridge for snacks isn't usually as long as your walk to the train and then on to the office. The NHS[55] advises that excessive sitting can affect your metabolism, blood pressure, blood sugar and cholesterol amongst other things. It's important to care for your physical health and a workout will help boost your fitness as well as provide a welcome break from work-related stress.

So how can you combat the holy trinity of working from home pitfalls: the bed, the fridge and the TV?

Schedule time for working out: a routine is key to ensure that you get the best out of your working day and you can incorporate exercise into this. Block out time in your diary to exercise, be it a gym class (online or in-person), a run or even dancing around to your favourite music.

Go for a walk: as you may no longer have to travel every day, try and create your own (much more pleasant) commute by going for a walk around the block in the morning. It will set you up for the day mentally plus it's healthier than doing a real commute.

Eat healthily: working from home means that you have more access to your fridge plus there's nobody to shame you if you decide to eat a cake on your own. To avoid emerging from working from home the size of the house, avoid junk food, plan healthy snacks (such as fruit or vegetables) and eat at regular times. It might be tempting to eat your meals at your desk but try to get up, prepare your meal in the kitchen and preferably eat it away from your desk. This way your brain will switch off from work temporarily, too.

Workouts to try at home

You might find yourself unable to get outside for a workout due to lack of time, space or funds. However, there are many routines available online, for free or paid, for you to do at home. You really have no excuse to skip your workout! You'll thank me later when those endorphins are pumping through your system.

FiiT: one of the leading go-to fitness apps with videos from the country's best instructors. From cardio, strength and rebalancing classes, there's something for everyone.

Couch to 5k: this NHS guided podcast will get you up and running in no time. Suitable for beginners.

For the 50+ market: Annie Deadman's *The 21 Day Blast Plan* is a three-week healthy eating and exercise programme that will get you into shape in no time. Alternatively, the National Institute of Ageing have a wide range of workout and stretching videos on YouTube.

GymCube: this online gym has over 700 classes for a £15 one-off payment. They also do live fitness classes which you can participate in – perfect if you want to interact with the instructor and see a friendly face.

Joe Wicks: the man who taught us how to get lean in fifteen. Buy his books or check out his Instagram page @ thebodycoach and YouTube channel @TheBodyCoachTV for an array of workouts.

Yoga with Adriene: the go-to free yoga series on YouTube, catering to all needs and situations. She has beginners' courses as well as more advanced sessions helpfully titled to help you find the right one for you. My favourite? Lower Back Love.

Low-impact, no-noise workouts: you may live in a block of flats and if you're bouncing around doing exercise classes, you're going to make yourself very unpopular very quickly. Check out the following YouTube channels for low-impact friendly workouts: TheBodyCoachTV, FitnessBlender and Zanna Van Dijk.

Desk exercises: you could do some simple desk exercises such as leg lifts and shoulder shrugs. If you're feeling a bit more energetic, why not try some star jumps or wall sits[56]? Check out the following YouTube channels for options: Forbes and SELF.

PART FOUR

IT'S NOT ALWAYS EASY

The positive stats about working from home are hard to ignore – from increasing your productivity to allowing you more flexibility in your life. But it can be tricky at times, especially at the start when you're figuring out a routine that works for you and potentially navigating the set-up with anyone you share your space with.

Academic Frances Hollis, who teaches at the Sir John Cass School of Art, Architecture and Design, did her doctoral thesis on working from home. She interviewed over a hundred remote workers[57] from all different walks of life. Even though the workers faced challenges and found working from home tough to adapt to initially, only six of the workers said that they wanted to return to working in an office after the study was completed. Everyone else loved working from home and the positive impact it had on the rest of their life; so, it's worth keeping at it.

Working with children

Chances are, if you're a parent right now or become a parent in the future, then you'll find yourself working from home whilst having to look after a child at some point. When trying to manage childcare and home working, it's inevitable that some days, work will win and other days, the children will win, but here's how to make the balance a little easier:

Set a schedule

This may be a schedule with your children, so they know what their routine is going to be for the day, as well as your work schedule. You may find that the Pomodoro Technique of working in twenty-five-minute blocks is useful (see p. 28) or you might work before your child wakes up, during their naptime and after bedtime. It might take some experimenting but it's worth discovering what works best for all of you.

Create an office space

Get creative with setting up your workspace so when you're in it, the children know that you're in work mode, perhaps by adding a sign for your office that says 'go' if you're available to talk to your children or 'stop' if you're busy (though obviously it goes without saying that if it's urgent, they can come into your office) or putting on a certain item of clothing when you're in work mode. Your children can help you make the sign or pick the clothing so they feel included. You may need to work around the house to keep an eye on them but if you can close the door, all the better.

Plan activities that don't need supervision

Try setting up activities that they can do on their own for a set amount of time whilst you work. Create a play box so they can keep themselves busy. Do not feel bad for letting them have screen time. Sometimes you have to do what you have to do to keep the peace. If you're worried about it, you can try to ensure that screen time is also educational. Try the following:

Science and maths

- Lightbot Coding
- The Human Body
- True or False Chemistry
- Elmo Loves 123s
- Squeebles Times Tables

Reading, spelling and phonics

- Duolingo
- Mr Thorne Does Phonics (YouTube)
- Teach Your Monster to Read
- Endless Alphabet
- Monkey Junior

Entertainment

- YouTube Kids
- DIY.org
- LEGO® Life
- Crossword Puzzles
- Toca Life: Vacation

Split jobs with others

If you have a partner, discuss how you can split looking after the children – potentially doing shifts – so you can get the focus you need. According to a study by University College London (UCL), women do sixteen hours[58] more around the house every week than men do, so try to make sure you split the housework as evenly as possible to make everyone's lives easier. If you need to arrange childcare, paid-for support is obviously one option – but it can be costly. You could share childcare with local families or alternatively, ask your friends and family whether they're able to pitch in. They could even turn their hand to virtual babysitting (assuming the children are of an appropriate age) where they keep watch over your children via Skype (for example, how about an art class? Watching a film together? Reading a story?) whilst you work.

Reward good behaviour

Make sure to praise your children if they respect your work boundaries and don't interrupt you when you're focusing on a certain task. Thank them for their help and reward them by spending some extra time with them doing an activity which they like.

Accept that nothing is perfect

You have to set realistic expectations as some days will be better than others. So don't beat yourself up if the day didn't go to plan, tomorrow is another day.

Working with others

More people share houses with others than ever before due to rising rents and the difficulty of getting on the housing ladder. According to the Institute of Fiscal Studies, house prices have risen at seven times the rate of wages in the UK and our chances of buying have halved over the past twenty years[59]. So, if you're also in a house share, like me, be it with your parents, your friends or your partner, here are my top tips to ensure you all work together as harmoniously as possible.

You might be the only person who works from home or there may be a few of you. Firstly, before agreeing to a house share, check with your new potential housemates that they're okay with you working from home. Some people aren't keen on it as they're worried about how this will impact the bills so it's best to have a chat about it up front. Once you know they're okay with it, you'll want to consider the following on a day-to-day basis.

Communicate: communicate clear boundaries so you understand what your housemates need and they know what you need in your workspace. And don't hog the best workspace or the best spot for the WiFi.

Treat them like colleagues: you wouldn't chat constantly to a colleague in the office, force them to look at memes every five minutes, take conference calls at your desk or eat smelly food, so don't do it at home. In my house, we work at the same table together but if one of us has to take a work call, we go to our bedrooms. Remember that your home, during certain hours, is a workspace and respect everyone's boundaries.

Keep your space tidy: it's easy to become a slob with your workspace but you share your space with others. At the end of the day, tidy up your workspace as not only will this help avoid tensions with your housemates/partner/family but it will help you switch from work to home mode.

Be conscious of bills: it may be tempting to have the heating on all day when you're working from home but if you share your space with others, discuss it with them first.

When I first went freelance, I had a conversation with my housemates about the bills and we agreed that in the colder months, I would have the heating on at certain times or would go and work in the library. When in doubt, layer up or get a hot water bottle on the go.

Get some space: as much as you love your housemates/ partner/family, factor in some alone time. Remember, you wouldn't be with colleagues at work 24/7 if you were in-house. Whether you go for a walk or schedule a quick phone call with a friend, a break will provide you with vital time-out.

What to do when you're having a bad day

We all have bad days. In fact, fitness app Freeletics did a survey of 2,000 people and discovered that on average, we have sixty bad days[60] a year. That's far too many days, if you ask me. The top contributing factors to a bad day are not enough sleep, financial worry, work-related stress, having plans fall through and a bad hair day (yes, really). And four out of five people blamed those bad days on work. Instead of letting yourself be consumed by bad feelings, try to look at it in a different light:

Treat yourself with compassion: it's easy to tell yourself that you're terrible at your job, but how about reminding yourself that you're doing the best you can in a potentially difficult and stressful situation.

Connect, connect, connect: you may find yourself working at home alone so pick up the phone or get outside. Interacting with someone else for a chat (even if it's just seeing another human being out shopping) will make you feel better and less alone. If you can rant down the phone to a sympathetic friend or colleague, so much the better.

Look after your body: you may be tempted to turn to your favourite junk food or a glass of something alcoholic. Before you do this, try a little workout, go for a walk or practice some mindfulness. According to Yale University and Oxford University, if you work out regularly, you'll have eighteen[61] fewer bad days a year than those who don't.

PART FIVE

MAKING WORKING FROM HOME WORK FOR YOU

Job flexibility is on the rise and it's only set to grow. There's been a 78 per cent increase in job posts globally that include the term 'job flexibility' (this can include options to work from home) since 2016[62] and well over two thirds of recruitment professionals agree that it's key to recruiting and retaining staff. Whether you're trying it for the first time or seasoned at working from home, or whether you're working on your own or managing a team, it's certainly an adjustment at the beginning. But there are a few easy ways to ensure you deliver results from day one.

Managers

How best to approach managing staff remotely? And how might you respond when a member of your team wants to change their working set-up and spend more time working flexibly?

Barbara Larson, a professor of management at Northeastern

University in Boston, explains that as a manager your role is to be the cheerleader of the team[63]. You should also try to set a good example when it comes to work-life balance by reminding your staff to work regular hours and take breaks. Provide them with the support they need as well as clear expectations, so they know what's required of them. You're going to need to be as flexible and sensitive as possible to your staff's needs.

Provide HR support

Your staff member might want to work from home a couple of days a week or month, or full time. ACAS[64] (the Advisory, Conciliation and Arbitration Service) advise that before you progress, you draw up an agreement with HR that covers your employee's schedule and individual needs (childcare, disability, health, etc.) so that they're working as effectively as possible for themselves as well as the business. Even if you work from home yourself, make sure you draw up an agreement too.

Introduce gradual transitions where possible

You don't want to thrust your employee straight in at the deep end. As Nicholas Bloom, a professor of economics at Stanford University, points out, 'you risk jeopardising the cohesion of your team'[65]. Trial one or two days a week if possible.

Build trust

One of the main reasons people aren't allowed to work from home is a lack of trust, according to Prithwiraj Choudhury[66], an associate professor in the Technology and Operations Management Unit at Harvard Business School. By communicating regularly with your staff and setting clear expectations, you'll begin to build trust amongst your team which will lead to better output. You should manage your staff on their outputs and not on the hours they spend at their desk. This promotes trust and also accountability.

Communicate

Most people thrive when they're part of a team. When you work in an office, you're constantly surrounded by others but when you're working from home, this is usually not the case. Communication is key, especially when it comes to maintaining team morale and productivity, so crank it up a notch. You can do this by kicking the day off with a call to run through the tasks that need to be completed that day, or round up the end of the working day with a check in. Psychologist Barbara Larson explains that face-to-face communication is far richer than talking on the phone so try to use video calls wherever possible to enhance human connection.

Strategist Arielle Tannenbaum explains that they have a system in place at Bustle[67] where new starters are paired with a different team member each week for a weekly call. This way they can get to know their team and share their goals and struggles when it comes to working from home.

Boost staff morale

Bloom suggests bringing office life into the home during working hours so people can have a chat with their colleagues, just as they would in the office kitchen, or arrange virtual work drinks (e-coffees are all the rage these days). Reward them when they hit certain performance targets with gift cards or time off.

Create a wellness support plan

The mental health charity Mind suggest setting up a wellness support plan[68] (available to download on their website) that will help you look after your staff's mental well-being as well as your own. Many companies now offer Employee Assistance Programmes (EAP) – an employer-funded benefit that provides contact with an independent adviser to confidentially discuss anything that is troubling them and is affecting their job performance – as a standard benefit so find out what is available at your company. A wellness support plan will itemise the elements that help your employee stay mentally healthy at work, what support you can provide them, any potentially stressful situations that may arise and warning signs you can look out for as their manager.

Monitor performance

As a manager responsible for those working from home, you need to understand that measurable work skills are going to look different[69]. Instead of focusing on more traditional work skills such as timekeeping, set an emphasis on outcome measures such as completing tasks and hitting targets.

Technology

Your role as a manager is to make sure that your team member has the necessary resources they need to do their job. Make sure you discuss with them what they require, such as a work laptop or other tools. Be proactive, so they don't have to raise it with you.

Employees

Asking your manager whether you can work from home can be nerve-wracking and there are a number of things you need to bear in mind before you proceed:

Why do you want to work from home?

Lots of people who work from home do it because it aligns with certain values or needs in their life. So, before you ask your manager whether it's a possibility for you, ask yourself why you want to do it. Is it because you want to spend more time with your family, save money or have a better work-life balance? Also consider how it will benefit the company as well. Remember that it's a give and take relationship.

Assess the situation

The second step is to do your homework and draw up a case to present to your manager. Does your role allow you to work from home? For example, you might already have meeting-free days during the week which means you can more easily work from home on those days. Perhaps you're an assistant whose job is more reactive to other's workload, so you'll need to discuss with them how working from home is going to be most efficient for your team. Will you receive the support you need from your company to work from home? How will your manager manage you remotely? These are all questions you need to ask yourself before you proceed with the next step. You should also prepare yourself for them to say no so you know how to respond and back your case up.

Know your rights

The Employment Rights Act (ERA) 1996 and the Flexible Working Regulations 2014 states that employees are allowed to make an application – a flexible working request – to their employer to change the terms and conditions of their role when it comes to the hours they work, when they do the work and where it is done. Each application needs to be considered on its merits. You can apply if you've worked for the company longer than twenty-six weeks[70], though do bear in mind that they're under no obligation to accept it, just to ensure they give it due and fair consideration. If your request is turned down, ask them to talk through their reasoning for declining it and how you could compromise or make an alternative proposal. If it's an outright refusal, you could escalate it to HR or to another manager.

How to ask your boss

You should always ask your boss about this in person, not via an email. Be sure to remind them of the benefits for both them and their staff: more productivity that in turn will generate more money, happier staff and higher staff retention. If your manager stands firm then you may have to consider how important working from home is for you and potentially look to work for a company that aligns more with your values.

Be flexible

It may take some time to be allowed to work from home full time, if that's what you want. Start by doing it one or two days a week, regularly checking in with your manager so you can see how it's working for the both of you as well as the rest of the team.

Demonstrate that you're serious

If your company is letting you work from home, step up to the plate and prove that you're serious about this change to your work environment. Suggest regular virtual meetings and phone calls, as well as key performance targets you want to hit so you're still a crucial part of the team. This is also a fantastic opportunity to be a role model for flexible working and to positively change the culture of your organisation. For example, you could be the first man in the company to work from home after having a child, empowering others to follow your lead and changing the culture in the office. Provide support to other colleagues and also give honest and open feedback to your line manager and HR.

Ask for the necessary support

Ask for the technology you may need for your job: software, computer, laptop. Check if your laptop needs to be encrypted as this will demonstrate that you understand the security implications of working from home. Make sure you undertake all necessary training and be proactive in your career development to make sure the business continues to see you as an active and committed employee.

What to do when working from home isn't working

Even though you've set everything up as best as you can, you may feel that working from home isn't working for you, or it might not be working for one of your team members. Below we explore the main issues that may arise, whether you're managing a team or are part of one.

For managers

Trust is a key factor when it comes to allowing staff members to work from home and you have to build this up over time. The more you trust your team, the happier they will be. That said, you may find yourself concerned that your employee isn't working as effectively as they could from home. Here's how you can help them:

- **Set clear parameters:** be sure to draw up a written agreement so that your employee is clear about what is expected of them and when. Targets will motivate your team, as will rewards when they hit them, so gently remind them of this if you're concerned.
- **Don't jump to conclusions:** try to be sensitive as your employee may be experiencing problems at home that you're unaware of. Think about what you can do to support them.

- **Consider whether flexible working works for your business:** if you've exhausted all of your options and don't think that it's working for your team, then you may have to consider whether flexible working is a practical option for your company.

For employees

- **Work-life balance:** you may find yourself in a situation in which your employer or team members assume that you're available to work all the time because you work from home. To avoid late night calls, set clear boundaries and communicate what your working hours are, perhaps in your email signature, so it's clear from the get-go.
- **Not enough support:** have your regular catch-ups with your manager started to slip? Do you feel lonely? Or perhaps you're not receiving the training you need? Bring up your concerns with your manager and team and suggest ways they can support you. By doing so, they'll get the best out of you, too.
- **Working from home isn't for you:** sometimes working from home isn't for everyone and it's okay to admit that to your boss. It takes sixty-six days[71] on average to form a new habit so I'd suggest trying to work your way through it for two or three months to see if you can find a routine that works for you.

- **Try and understand why it's not working for you:** is this because you don't think you're receiving enough support or you're not as productive as you thought you would be? Explore these questions with your manager as well as friends and family.

CONCLUSION

WHAT THE FUTURE HOLDS

I hope by this point, I've shown you that working from home can be genuinely beneficial for all aspects of your life, as well as your business or your employer's business. The world of working is constantly evolving, and the future is bright for those who want to work from home.

Technology will lead the charge and, as society changes, working from home will become much more the norm. Dave Nevogt, CEO of Hubstaff, a remote time and team management company, believes that businesses are catching on to how positive working from home can be for them 'likely because they've experienced the benefits of greater productivity, less wasted time and lower overheads first hand.'[72]

The younger generations are becoming digital nomads who choose to embrace a technology-enabled lifestyle that allows them to work anywhere in the world. According to MBO's annual State of Independence in America survey, at the end of 2017 there were 4.8 million digital nomads in the world and over 17 million people aspire to be so in the future[73].

As for older generations, childcare could look radically different in the future. As more parents start to work from home, perhaps the cost of childcare may change as some parents might not need their children to be in childcare all day. And of course, we mustn't forget the impact this will have on our environment, especially when it comes to keeping pollution down. The positive possibilities are endless.

Personally, working from home has changed my life for the better and I've found that my professional values are more in line with my personal values which makes for a great motivator. I can work creatively and effectively with different teams across the globe, all from the comfort of my home, whilst also having a better work-life balance. Like you, I'm a typical home worker who had to muddle their way through it at the beginning but I got there, and I'm confident you can, too.

Now, more than ever, we have a choice about how we want to work so be open to change and embrace it. See you at home.

FURTHER RESOURCES

Useful tools

- **Time management tools:** use timers such as Toggl (web), Stand Up! The Work Break Timer (app), Focus Booster (app and web) or TomatoTimer (web) to track your time.
- **Site blockers:** Freedom, StayFocusd and SelfControl are apps available for your devices that block distracting websites and apps so you can remain focused on the task on hand instead of watching funny cat videos.
- **Video conferencing:** make your virtual meetings as pain-free as possible with Zoom, Google Hangouts and Skype.
- **Chat online:** sometimes you need an instant response so turn to Slack and Teams for virtual messaging.
- **Team management:** set up an easy and effective way for you to manage your team's work in one place with Asana, Trello and Monday.com.

Books to read

Remote: Office Not Required by David Heinemeier Hansson and Jason Fried: remote working is the future and this call of action will explain how.

Work Together Anywhere: A Handbook on Working Remotely – Successfully – for Individuals, Teams, and Managers by Lisette Sutherland and Kirsten Janene-Nelson: this blueprint will help you optimise success not only for yourself but for your team as well.

The Multi-Hyphen Method by Emma Gannon: in this practical book, author-podcaster Emma Gannon encourages you to think about your work-life balance in a new way and even turn your side-hustle into a career.

The Freelance Bible by Alison Grade: have you decided to go freelance but don't know where to begin? Award-winning entrepreneur Alison Grade is here to guide you through it.

Podcasts to listen to

The Productivityist Podcast: hosted by productivity strategist Mike Vardy, this podcast will discuss the tips and tricks you need to take your productivity to the next level.

The Tim Ferriss Show: bestselling author of international bestseller *The 4-Hour Workweek*, entrepreneur Tim Ferriss chats to world-class performers to discover the tools they use to achieve success.

WorkLife with Adam Grant: organisational psychologist Adam Grant delves into the minds of some of the world's most unusual professionals to see what makes them tick and how they've become so successful.

Freelance Feels: a well-being podcast by lifestyle journalist Jenny Stallard who speaks to others about how they work best remotely, as well as the ups and downs they face.

Creative Rebels: David Speed and Adam Brazier, founders of Graffiti Life and Parlour Tattoo, chat to creatives who have rebelled against the 9-5 to find a work set-up that works best for them.

The High Performance Podcast: get a glimpse into the lives of high-achieving performers and learn about the non-negotiable behaviours they employ to ensure that they're at the top of their game.

ENDNOTES

1. **By the end of 2019, one in five of us around the globe were already working from home**

   Jude Gonzalez, 'Working from home could make your happier – especially if you're married', Phys (27 February 2018), https://phys.org/news/2018-02-home-happier-youre.html

2. **There's been a 74 per cent increase in those who work from home since 2008**

   Rory Claydon and Kate McGough, 'I turn off the doorbell when I work from home', BBC (7 May 2019), https://www.bbc.co.uk/news/business-48180804

3. **Over half of the respondents said flexibility was the greatest advantage for them when it comes to working from home**

   Rory Claydon and Kate McGough, 'I turn off the doorbell when I work from home', BBC (7 May 2019), https://www.bbc.co.uk/news/business-48180804

4. **Eight out of ten businesses said that flexible working has made their business more productive**

   International Workplace Group (IWG), 'The IWG Global

Workspace Survey', IWG (March 2019), https://assets.regus.com/pdfs/iwg-workplace-survey/iwg-workplace-survey-2019.pdf

5.   ... described working from home as having as much potential as a driverless car

TedXTalks, 'Go ahead, tell your boss you are working from home – Nicholas Bloom, TEDx STANFORD' (22 May 2017), https://www.youtube.com/watch?v=oiUyyZPIHyY

6.   The average officer worker spends over £6 a day on lunch

Jack Peat, 'One in three Brits face "déjà-food" on a daily basis', *Independent* (21 September 2018), https://www.independent.co.uk/news/health/one-in-three-brits-food-envy-a8547201.html

7.   In America, on average, a worker can spend between $2,000-5000 a year on getting to and from the workplace

Marissa Perino, 'Here's what the average person spends on their commute annually in every state', Business Insider (18 July 2019), https://www.businessinsider.com/average-spending-on-commute-how-much-money-2019-7?r=US&IR=T

8.   London, Sydney, Dublin, the top three most expensive commutes in the world

'The Global Public Transport Index', Globehunters (Updated 17 July 2019) https://www.globehunters.us/blog/the-global-public-transport-index.htm

9.   The average UK worker spends 400 days of theirs lives commuting

'UK commuters will spend over £135,000 by the time they retire', Totaljobs (accessed 26 March 2020), https://www.totaljobs.com/insidejob/uk-commuters-will-spend-over-135000-by-the-time-they-retire/

10.   The average cost for a square foot of office space in London, for example, costs seventy pounds a month

Statista Research Department, 'Cost of office rent in London in the second quarter 2019, by area' (18 February 2020), https://www.statista.com/statistics/873480/london-office-cost-of-rent/

11. In Manchester it [a square foot of office space] costs about thirty pounds a month

'Manchester watch: Manchester offices', Savills (19 November 2018), https://www.savills.co.uk/research_articles/229130/270333-0/market-watch--manchester-offices---november-2018

12. **The average cost of hiring a new employee is £11,000**

International Workplace Group (IWG), 'The IWG Global Workspace Survey', IWG (March 2019), https://assets.regus.com/pdfs/iwg-workplace-survey/iwg-workplace-survey-2019.pdf

13. **In Poland, 92 per cent of employers use this strategy [flexible working as recruitment tool]**

International Workplace Group (IWG), 'The IWG Global Workspace Survey', IWG (March 2019), https://assets.regus.com/pdfs/iwg-workplace-survey/iwg-workplace-survey-2019.pdf

14. **Over a million disabled people work from home**

Frances O'Grady, 'Working from home is on the rise – but why so slow?', Trade Union Congress (17 May 2019), https://www.tuc.org.uk/blogs/working-home-rise-why-so-slow

15. **Almost twice as many men as women who work from home**

Frances O'Grady, 'Working from home is on the rise – but why so slow?', Trade Union Congress (17 May 2019), https://www.tuc.org.uk/blogs/working-home-rise-why-so-slow

16. **Those from a BAME background are less likely to be able to work from home compared to white workers – 4.3 per cent to 6.5 per cent**

Frances O'Grady, 'Working from home is on the rise – but why so slow?', Trade Union Congress (17 May 2019), https://www.tuc.org.uk/blogs/working-home-rise-why-so-slow

17. **BAME millennials are 47 per cent more likely to be on a zero-hours contract**

     Caroline Davies, 'BAME millennials have less stable working lives than their white peers', *Guardian* (2 March 2020), https://www.theguardian.com/money/2020/mar/02/bame-millennials-less-stable-work-lives-than-white-peers

18. **Decisions may be disproportionality made on the basis of job title hierarchy**

     Frances O'Grady, 'Working from home is on the rise – but why so slow?', Trade Union Congress (17 May 2019), https://www.tuc.org.uk/blogs/working-home-rise-why-so-slow

19. **Managers are twice as likely to work at home compared to the average employee**

     Frances O'Grady, 'Working from home is on the rise – but why so slow?', Trade Union Congress (17 May 2019), https://www.tuc.org.uk/blogs/working-home-rise-why-so-slow

20. **Companies in the bottom quartile for both gender and cultural diversity are less likely to achieve above-average profitability**

     'Delivering through diversity', McKinsey & Company (January 2018), https://www.mckinsey.com/~/media/McKinsey/Business%20Functions/Organization/Our%20Insights/Delivering%20through%20diversity/Delivering-through-diversity_full-report.ashx

21. **Over two thirds of those who took part said that working from home has allowed them to be happier**

     Brie Weller Reynolds, 'FlexJobs 2018 Annual Survey: Workers Believe a Flexible or Remote Job Can Help Save Money, Reduce Stress, and More', FlexJobs (8 September 2018), https://www.flexjobs.com/blog/post/flexjobs-2018-annual-survey-workers-believe-flexible-remote-job-can-help-save-money-reduce-stress-more

22. **This productivity gain could add $1.3 billion to the US economy every year**

Kristen Senz, 'How companies benefit when employees work remotely', Harvard Business School (29 July 2019), https://hbswk.hbs.edu/item/how-companies-benefit-when-employees-work-remotely

23. **Job satisfaction declines with commute time**

Jeremy Allen, 'Commuting has Multiple Impacts on Employee Wellbeing', University of the West of England (27 October 2017), https://blogs.uwe.ac.uk/research-business-innovation/commuting-has-multiple-impacts-on-employee-wellbeing/

24. **Those who work from home are only sick 1.8 days a year compared to workers in an office who take an average of 3.1 sick days**

Sophie Smith, 'Seven reasons why home working is the future', *Telegraph* (15 November 2018), https://www.telegraph.co.uk/education-and-careers/2017/07/24/seven-reasons-home-working-future/

25. **The car is the most used mode of transport for commuting**

'British workers spend 492 days of their lives travelling into work', Lloyds Bank (6 September 2019), https://www.lloydsbankinggroup.com/Media/Press-Releases/2019-press-releases/lloyds-bank/british-workers-spend-492-days-of-their-lives-travelling-into-work/

26. **In London, a car costs the NHS and society £8,000 in health bills due to air pollution and nearly £6bn for the country**

Josh Gabbatiss, 'Each car in London costs NHS and society £8,000 due to air pollution, report finds', *Independent* (6 June 2018), https://www.independent.co.uk/environment/cars-air-pollution-cost-nhs-vans-vehicles-health-bills-lung-disease-a8384806.html

27. **If a quarter of the journeys were spent walking or cycling, then the nation could save over £1.1bn**

Josh Gabbatiss, 'Each car in London costs NHS and society

£8,000 due to air pollution, report finds', *Independent* (6 June 2018), https://www.independent.co.uk/environment/cars-air-pollution-cost-nhs-vans-vehicles-health-bills-lung-disease-a8384806.html

28. **Productivity increases by well over 10 per cent when people work from home**

    Nicholas Bloom, James Liang, John Roberts and Zhichun Jenny Ying, 'Does working from home work? Evidence from a Chinese experiment' (2014), https://nbloom.people.stanford.edu/sites/g/files/sbiybj4746/f/wfh.pdf

29. **On average, those who worked from home worked an extra 1.4 days a month and 16 days a year**

    'The benefits of working from home', Airtasker (updated 9 September 2019), https://www.airtasker.com/blog/the-benefits-of-working-from-home/

30. **A quarter of workers said they had pain caused by a poor home office set-up and this impacted their productivity**

    Ashleigh Webber, 'Workers spend 67 days a year sitting at a desk', Personnel Today (17 October 2018), https://www.personneltoday.com/hr/staff-spend-67-sedentary-working-days/

31. **The average office worker spends 1,700 hours at their desk a year**

    Grant Bailey, 'Office workers spend 1,700 hours a year in front of a computer screen', *Independent* (23 July 2018), https://www.independent.co.uk/news/uk/home-news/office-workers-screen-headaches-a8459896.html

32. **Matthew Devoe, an American chiropractor, explains that a bad set-up will likely result in 'tech neck'**

    Suzy Weiss, 'Working from home? Here's how to make your setup more ergonomic', *New York Post* (17 March 2020), https://nypost.com/2020/03/17/working-from-home-heres-how-to-make-your-setup-more-ergonomic/

33. **We know that sitting all day isn't good for our bodies so how about trying a standing desk?**

   'Office workers of England – stand up for your health!, NHS (2 June 2015), https://www.nhs.uk/news/lifestyle-and-exercise/office-workers-of-england-stand-up-for-your-health/

34. **The brain works better when we move, instead of spending hours hunched over our desk, and our productivity increases as a result**

   Greg Wells, '3 Ways Walking Away From Your Desk Makes You Smarter', Entrepreneur (28 September 2016), https://www.entrepreneur.com/article/281967

35. **Placing a pillow on your chair, be it a foldable chair or a dining table one, will elevate you and relieve pressure on your spine**

   Daniel Varghese, 'Building an Ergonomic Home Office: How to Fix Your WFH Posture, *GQ* (25 March 2020), https://www.gq.com/story/tips-for-an-ergonomic-home-office

36. **To avoid eye strain, reduce the glare of outside light by drawing the curtains or blinds, and indoor lighting by using a desk or floor lamp instead of harsh overhead lighting**

   'Computer Eye Strain', Specsavers (accessed 2 April 2020), https://www.specsavers.co.uk/eye-health/computer-eye-strain-symptoms-and-solutions

37. **You should position your computer screen at least 51cm away from your eyes**

   'The Ergonomic Equation', Ergotron (accessed 2 April 2020), https://www.ergotron.com/en-gb/ergonomics/ergonomic-equation

38. **Four out of ten workers in the UK still say that a lack of necessary technology provided by their employer prevents them from working from home as often as they'd like**

   International Workplace Group (IWG), 'The IWG Global Workspace Survey', IWG (March 2019), https://assets.regus.com/

pdfs/iwg-workplace-survey/iwg-workplace-survey-2019.pdf

39. **Almost half of them reported using headphones to avoid distractions**

    Robin Madell, 'Surprising Results About Wearing Headphones at Work and Productivity', FlexJobs (16 December 2018), https://www.flexjobs.com/blog/post/surprising-results-about-wearing-headphones-at-work-productivity/

40. **Professor Kelly was gatecrashed by his children during a live interview**

    BBC, 'Prof Robert Kelly and family – the full interview, BBC News (14 March 2017), https://www.bbc.co.uk/news/av/world-asia-39274662/prof-robert-kelly-and-family-the-full-interview

41. **Interruptions and being talked over are two of the biggest meeting challenges**

    Meredith Hart, 'Video conferencing etiquette: 10 tips for a successful video conference', OWLLabs (25 March 2020), https://www.owllabs.com/blog/video-conferencing-etiquette

42. **Only a measly 3 per cent of us are any good at multitasking**

    Jason M. Watson and David L. Strayer, 'Supertaskers: Profiles in extraordinary multitasking ability', *Psychonomic Bulletin & Review* (2010), http://www.psych.uncc.edu/pagoolka/seminar/PBR2010p479.pdf

43. **Kristen Shockley suggests 'psychological segues' such as a coffee or a workout to close your working day**

    Bryan Lufkin, 'Coronavirus: How to work from home, the right way', BBC (13 March 2020), https://www.bbc.com/worklife/article/20200312-coronavirus-covid-19-update-work-from-home-in-a-pandemic

44. **We make the mistake of writing everything down without any structure**

Bianca Barratt, 'How to write a to do list that you'll actually stick to', Forbes (30 January 2019), https://www.forbes.com/sites/biancabarratt/2019/01/30/how-to-write-a-to-do-list-that-youll-actually-stick-to/#336357cd279e

45. **There are four types of people in the world, depending on their sleep habits**

Rich Bellis, 'How to design your ideal workday based on your sleep habits', Fast Company (26 November 2017), https://www.fastcompany.com/40491564/how-to-design-your-ideal-workday-based-on-your-sleep-habits

46. **We should spend at least twenty minutes focusing on one task instead of flitting between many different ones**

Eyal Ophir, Clifford Nass, and Anthony D. Wagner, 'Cognitive control in media multitaskers', Proceedings of the National Academy of Sciences of the United States of America (PNAS) (15 September 2009), https://www.pnas.org/content/106/37/15583.full

47. **You could create a smart playlist that changes songs at set intervals**

Alexandra Franzen, '10 simple ways to become a better writer', The Muse (accessed 25 March 2020), https://www.themuse.com/advice/10-simple-ways-to-become-a-better-writer

48. **Wearing more formal clothing can boost your abstract thinking**

Matthew Hutson and Toni Rodriguez, 'Dress for success: how clothes influence our performance', Scientific American (1 January 2016), https://www.scientificamerican.com/article/dress-for-success-how-clothes-influence-our-performance/

49. **Wearing a doctor's coat can help you be more focused**

Hajo Adam and Adam D. Galinsky, 'Enclothed cognition', Journal of Experimental Social Psychology – volume 48, Issue 4 (July 2012), https://www.sciencedirect.com/science/article/abs/pii/S0022103112000200

50. **Psychologists have identified three key elements that sustain your motivation**

Daisy Yuhas, 'Three Critical Elements Sustain Motivation, *Scientific American* (1 November 2012), https://www.scientificamerican.com/article/three-critical-elements-sustain-motivation/

51. **Businesses are using flexible working as a way to improve their employees' work-life balance**

International Workplace Group (IWG), 'The IWG Global Workspace Survey', IWG (March 2019), https://assets.regus.com/pdfs/iwg-workplace-survey/iwg-workplace-survey-2019.pdf

52. **Participants' biggest struggle with working from home was being unable to unplug from work**

'State of Remote Work: 2019', Buffer (accessed 26 March 2020), https://buffer.com/state-of-remote-work-2019

53. **Working from home can also mean three hours of extra childcare**

'Germany: Flexible working conditions lead to overtime, study shows', DW Academie (accessed 25 March 2020), https://www.dw.com/en/germany-flexible-working-conditions-lead-to-overtime-study-shows/a-47771436

54. **Loneliness was the second-most reported challenge after unplugging from work**

'State of Remote Work: 2019', Buffer (accessed 26 March 2020), https://buffer.com/state-of-remote-work-2019

55. **Excessive sitting can affect your metabolism, blood pressure, blood sugar and cholesterol**

'Why we should sit less', NHS (last reviewed 22 November 2019), https://www.nhs.uk/live-well/exercise/why-sitting-too-much-is-bad-for-us/

56. **Why not try some star jumps or wall sits?**

Emily Cooper, '6 simple daily desk exercises', Posture People (13

March 2020), https://www.posturepeople.co.uk/6-simple-daily-desk-exercises/

57. **Even though the workers faced challenges and found working from home tough to adapt to initially, only six of the workers said that they wanted to return to working in an office after the study was completed**

Dale Berning Sawa, 'Extreme loneliness or the perfect balance? How to work from home and stay healthy', *Guardian* (25 March 2019), https://www.theguardian.com/lifeandstyle/2019/mar/25/extreme-loneliness-or-the-perfect-balance-how-to-work-from-home-and-stay-healthy

58. **Women do 16 hours more around the house every week than men do**

Sabrina Barr, 'Women still do majority of household chores, study finds', *Independent* (26 July 2019), https://www.independent.co.uk/life-style/women-men-household-chores-domestic-house-gender-norms-a9021586.html

59. **House prices have risen at seven times the rate of wages in the UK and our chances of buying have halved over the past twenty years**

Zoe Beaty, 'Generation rent: Stylist investigates the rising popularity of houseshares', *Stylist* (accessed 25 March 2020), https://www.stylist.co.uk/life/houseshares-pros-cons-having-flatmates-generation-rent/258346

60. **We have sixty bad days a year**

Tyler Schmall, 'Having a bad day? The average American has 60 per year, study says', FOX News (14 February 2018), https://www.foxnews.com/lifestyle/having-a-bad-day-the-average-american-has-60-per-year-study-says

61. **If you work out regularly then you're more likely to have eighteen bad days fewer a year than those who don't**

Ruqayyah Moynihan, 'Exercise is more important for your mental health than money, Yale and Oxford research suggests', Business Insider (11 February 2020), https://www.businessinsider.com/exercise-makes-you-happier-than-money-says-yale-and-oxford-study-2019-4?r=US&IR=T

62. **There's been a 78 per cent increase in job posts globally that include the term 'job flexibility' since 2016**

    'LinkedIn Releases 2019 Global Talent Trends Report', LinkedIn (28 January 2019), https://news.linkedin.com/2019/January/linkedin-releases-2019-global-talent-trends-report

63. **As a manager your role is to be the cheerleader of the team**

    Bryan Lufkin, 'Coronavirus: How to work from home, the right way', BBC (13 March 2020), https://www.bbc.com/worklife/article/20200312-coronavirus-covid-19-update-work-from-home-in-a-pandemic

64. **Draw up an agreement with HR that covers your employee's schedule and individual needs**

    'Working from home', the Advisory, Conciliation and Arbitration Service (ACAS) (accessed 26 March 2020), https://www.acas.org.uk/working-from-home

65. **Introduce gradual transitions where possible**

    Billy Murphy Jr., 'A Stanford Professor Says Working From Home Makes You Happier and More Efficient. There's Just 1 Catch', Inc. (14 December 2017), https://www.inc.com/bill-murphy-jr/people-who-work-from-home-are-happier-more-efficient-according-to-this-fascinating-study-theres-only-1-catch.html

66. **One of the main reasons people aren't allowed to work from home is a lack of trust**

    'The Benefits Of Working (Very) Remotely', Forbes (12 August 2019), https://www.forbes.com/sites/hbsworkingknowledge/2019/

08/12/the-benefits-of-working-very-remotely/#123b258953c0

67. New starters are paired with a different team member each week
     for a weekly call

     Arielle Tannenbaum, 'Remote workers share how they conquer
     loneliness', Fast Company (26 June 2018), https://www.fastcompany.
     com/40589281/remote-workers-share-how-they-conquer-loneliness

68. **The mental health charity Mind suggest setting up a wellness
     support plan**

     Emma Mamo, 'Coronavirus: supporting yourself and your team',
     Mind (accessed 26 March 2020), https://www.mind.org.uk/
     workplace/mental-health-at-work/coronavirus-supporting-yourself-
     and-your-team/

69. **As a manager responsible for those working from home, you
     need to understand that measurable work skills are going to look
     different**

     'A means to many ends', Age UK (September 2012) https:/
     /www.ageuk.org.uk/globalassets/age-uk/documents/reports-
     and-publications/reports-and-briefings/active-communities/
     rb_sept12_a_means_to_many_ends_older_workers_experiences_
     of_flexible_working.pdf

70. **You can apply [to work from home] if you've worked for the
     company longer than twenty-six weeks**

     'Flexible Working – changes in the law – June 2014', Pothecary
     Witham Weld Solicitors (accessed 26 March 2020), https:/
     /www.pwwsolicitors.co.uk/2013-07-01-14-12-06/individuals/
     128-flexible-working-changes-in-the-law-june-2014

71. **It takes sixty-six days on average to form a new habit**

     Roger Dobson, 'It takes 66 days to form a habit', *Telegraph*
     (18 July 2009) https://www.telegraph.co.uk/news/health/news/
     5857845/It-takes-66-days-to-form-a-habit.html

72. **Businesses are catching on to how positive working from home can be for them**

'State of Remote Work: 2019', Buffer (accessed 26 March 2020), https://buffer.com/state-of-remote-work-2019

73. **At the end of 2017 there were 4.8 million digital nomads in the world and over 17 million people aspire to be so in the future**

'Digital Nomadism: A Rising Trend', MBO Partners (2018), https://s29814.pcdn.co/wp-content/uploads/2019/02/StateofIndependence-ResearchBrief-DigitalNomads.pdf

NOTES